FLOWER POWER!
A BOOK THAT MAKES SCENTS

For Ellie,
I hope you
enjoy hearing
the story and
looking at
the colors!
Love,
Aunt
Erin

**Written and Illustrated by
Erin Muñoz**

For my Little Xela.

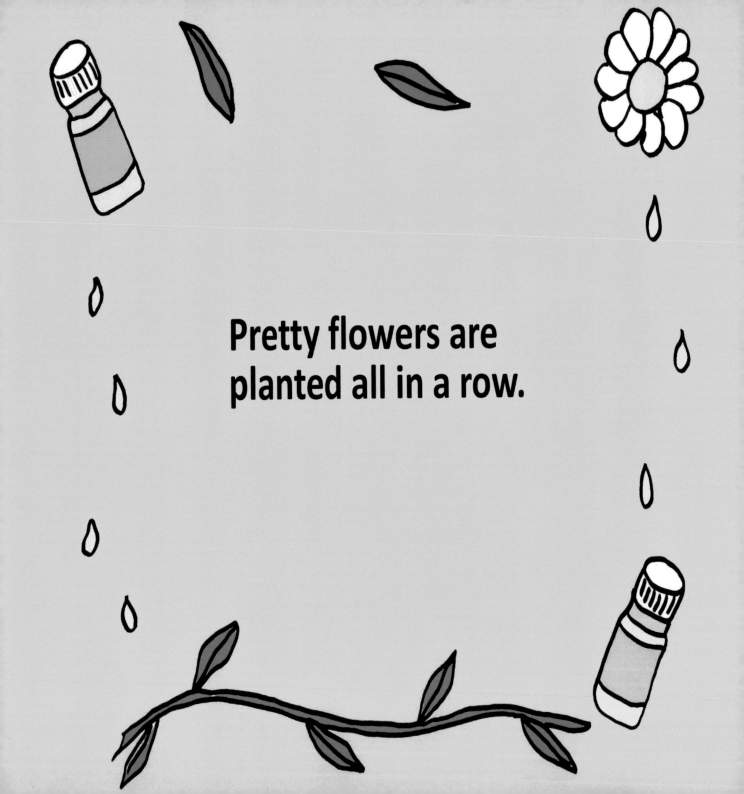

Pretty flowers are
planted all in a row.

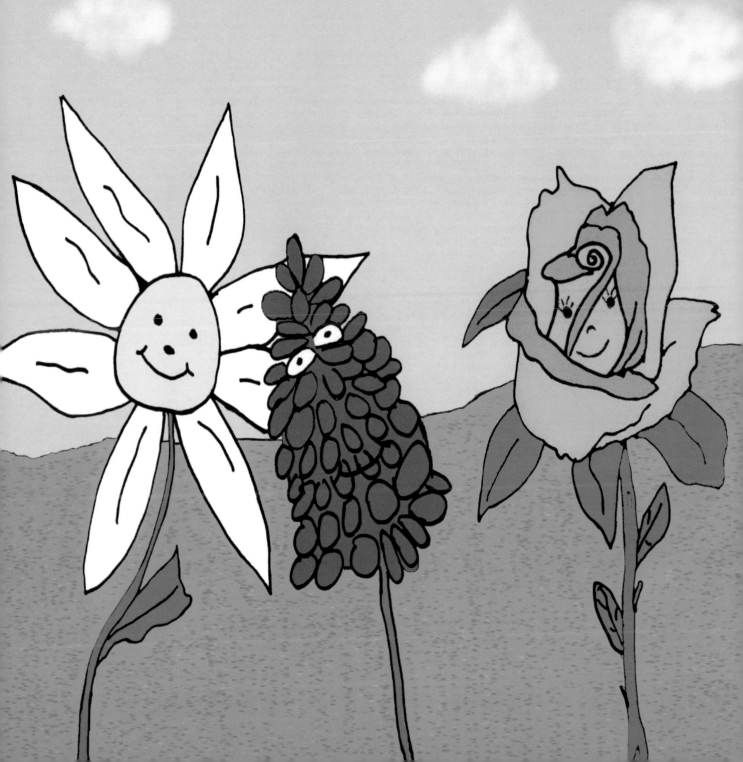

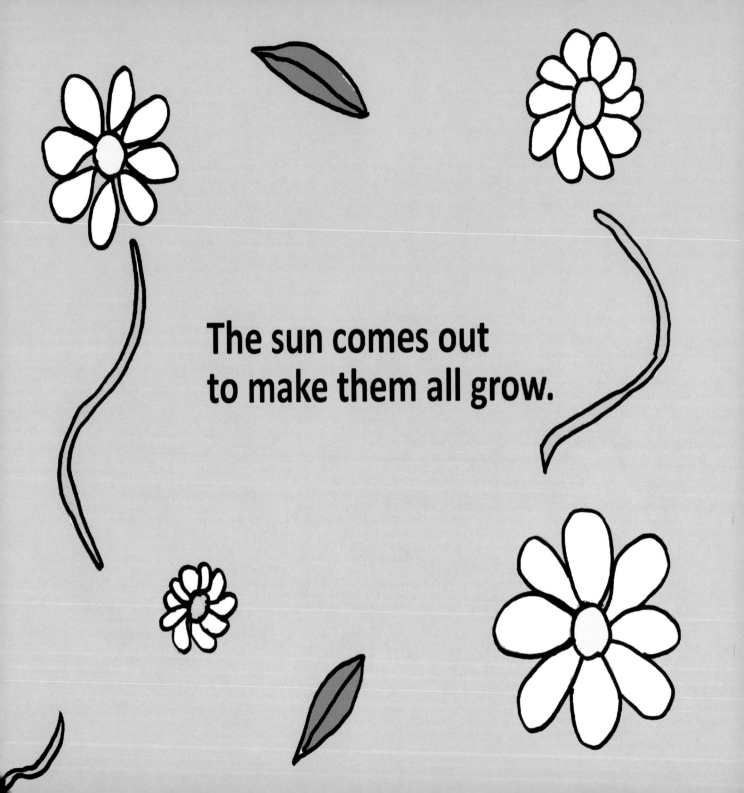

The sun comes out
to make them all grow.

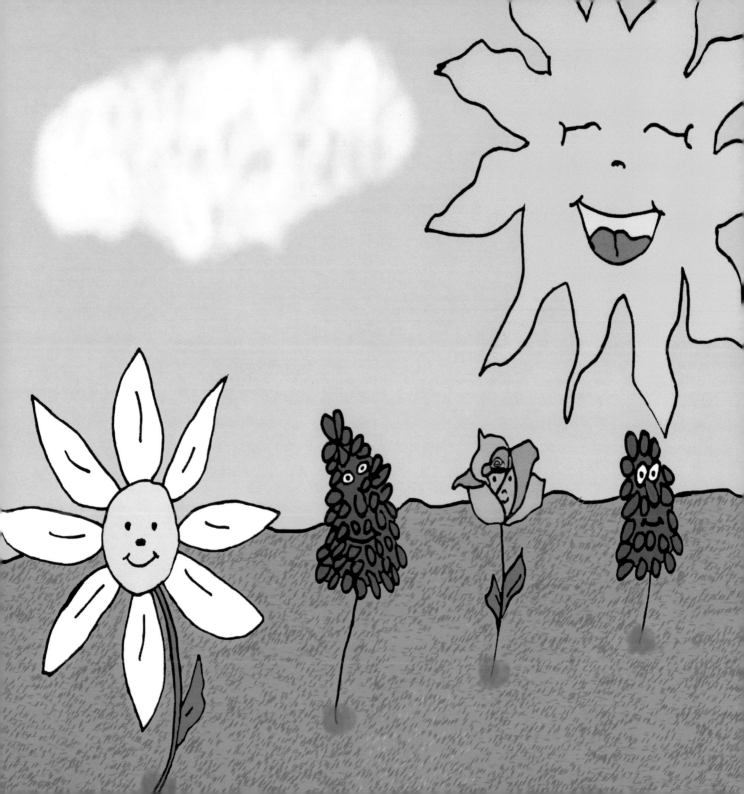

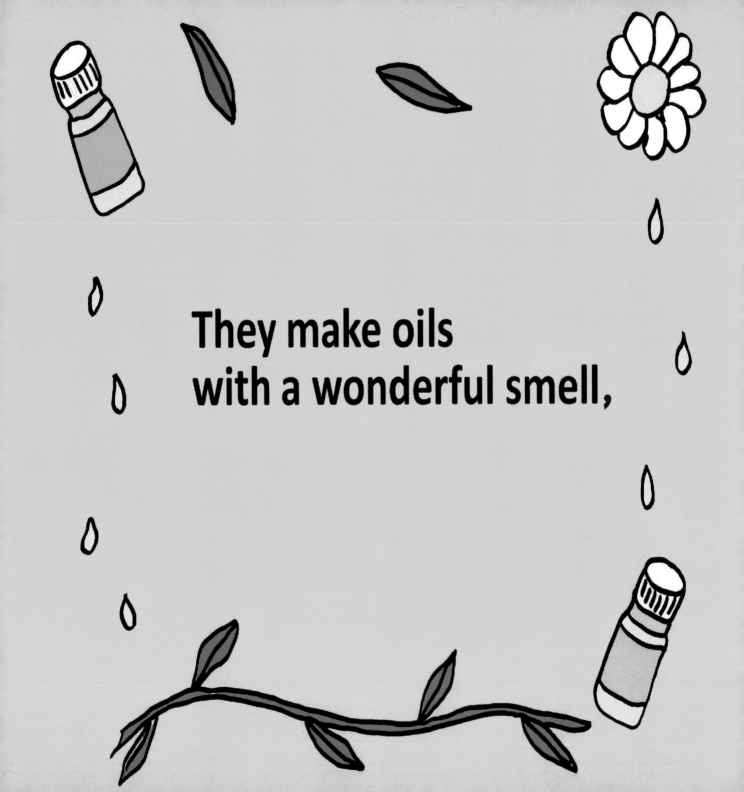

They make oils
with a wonderful smell,

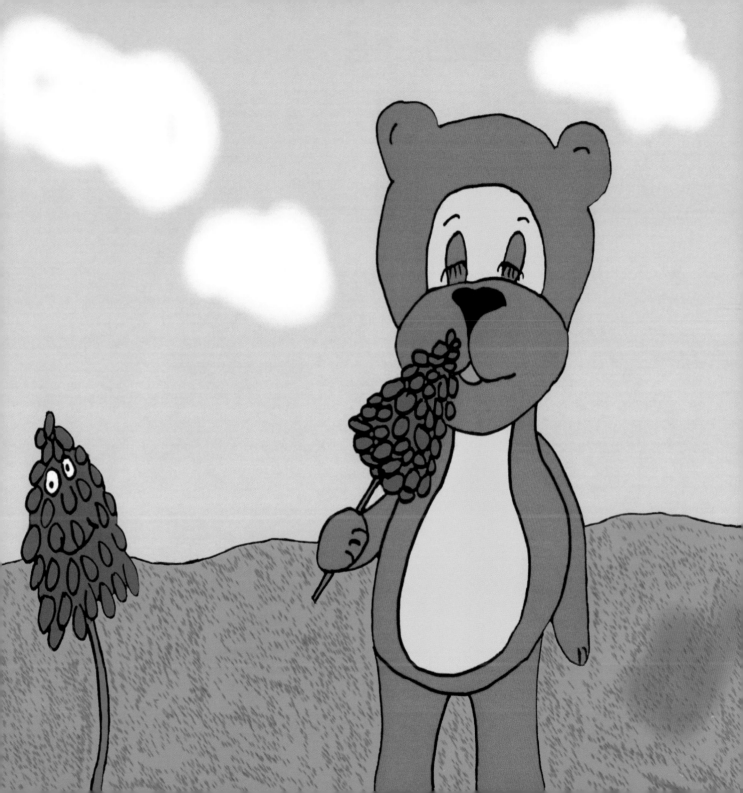

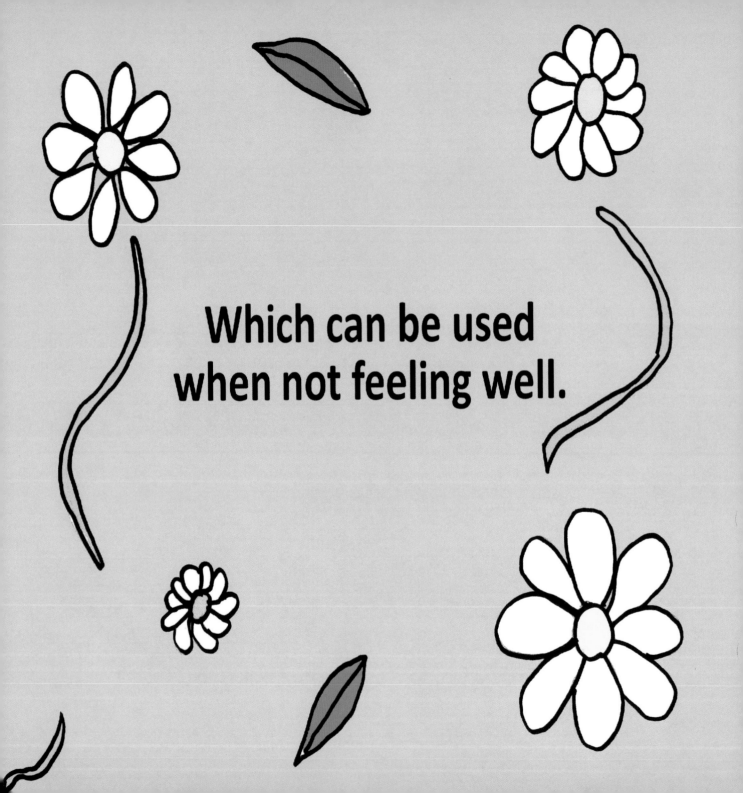

Which can be used
when not feeling well.

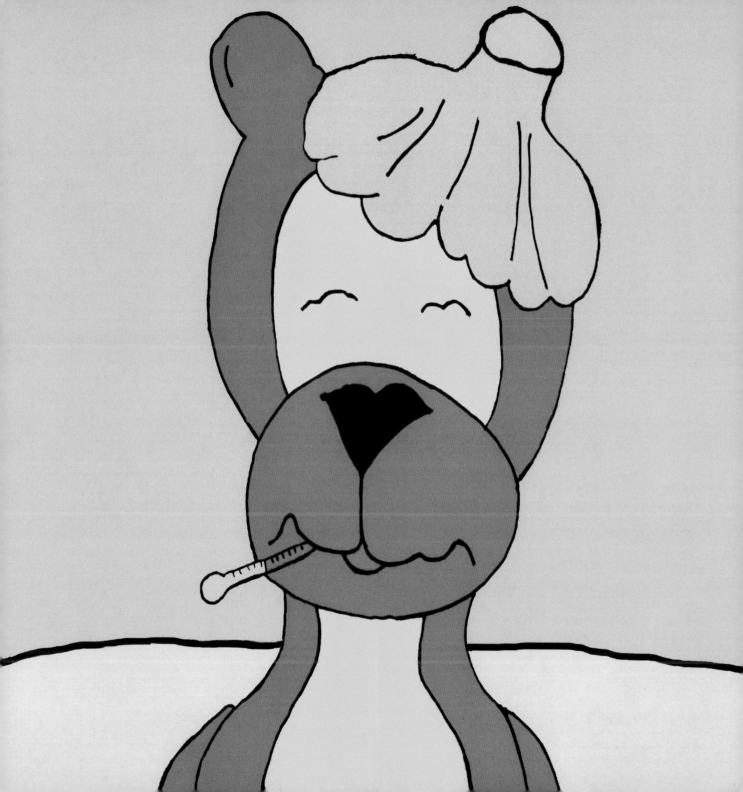

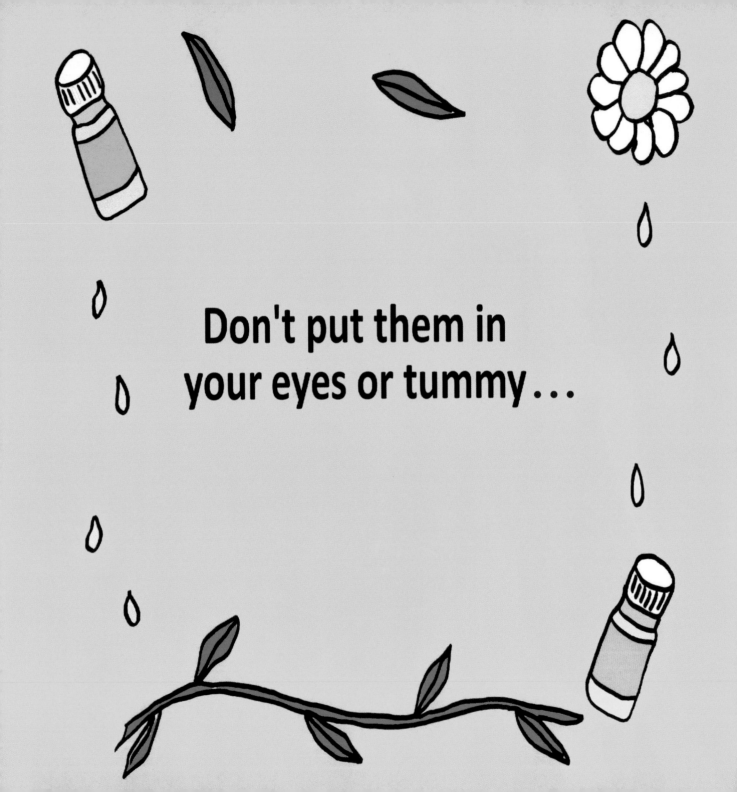

Don't put them in
your eyes or tummy...

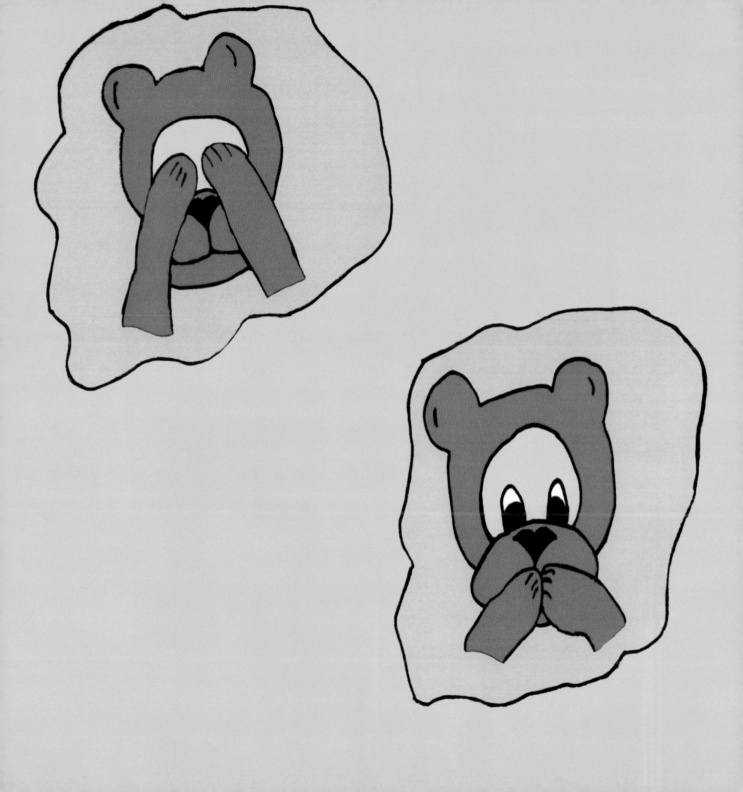

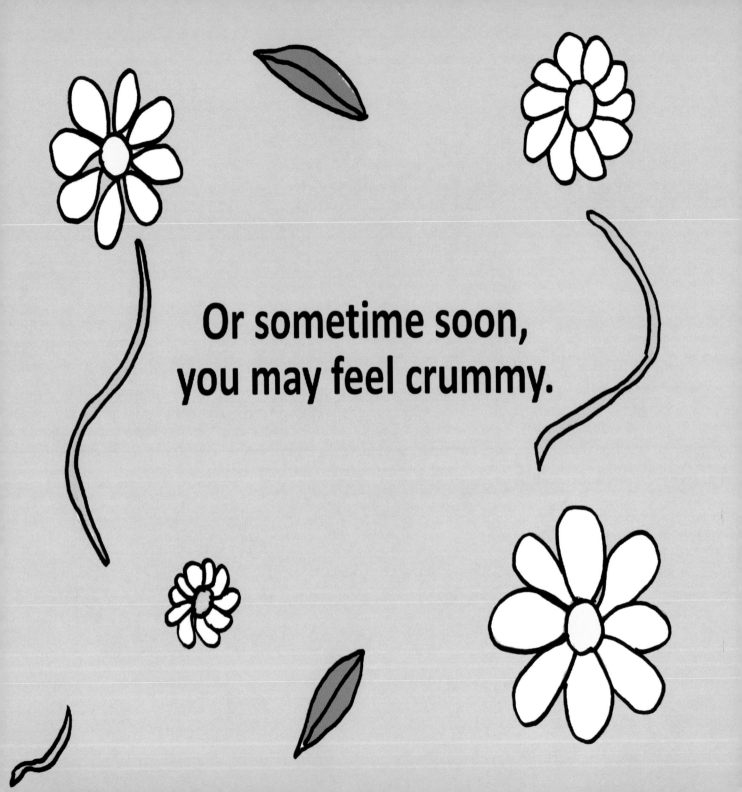

Or sometime soon,
you may feel crummy.

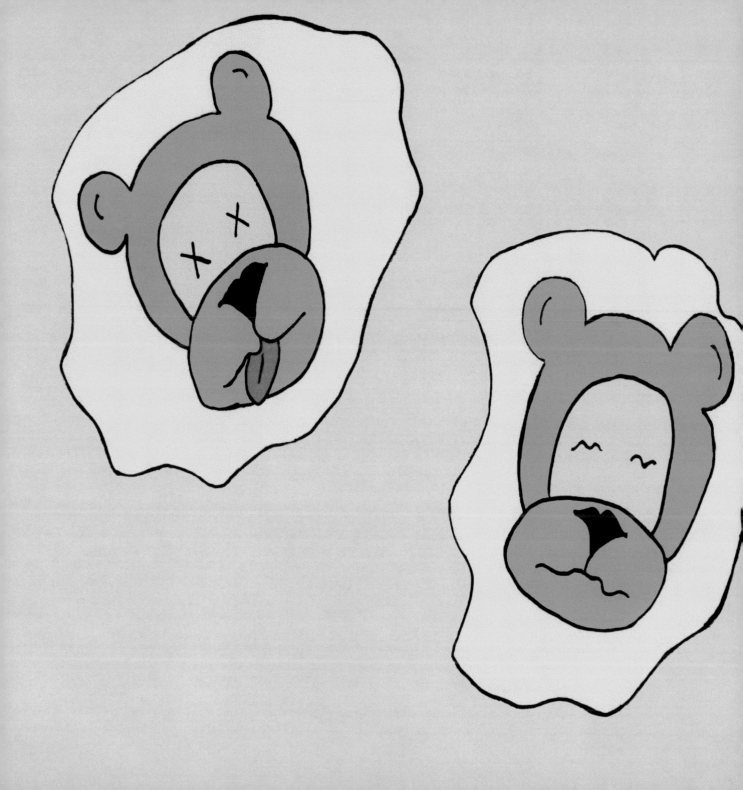

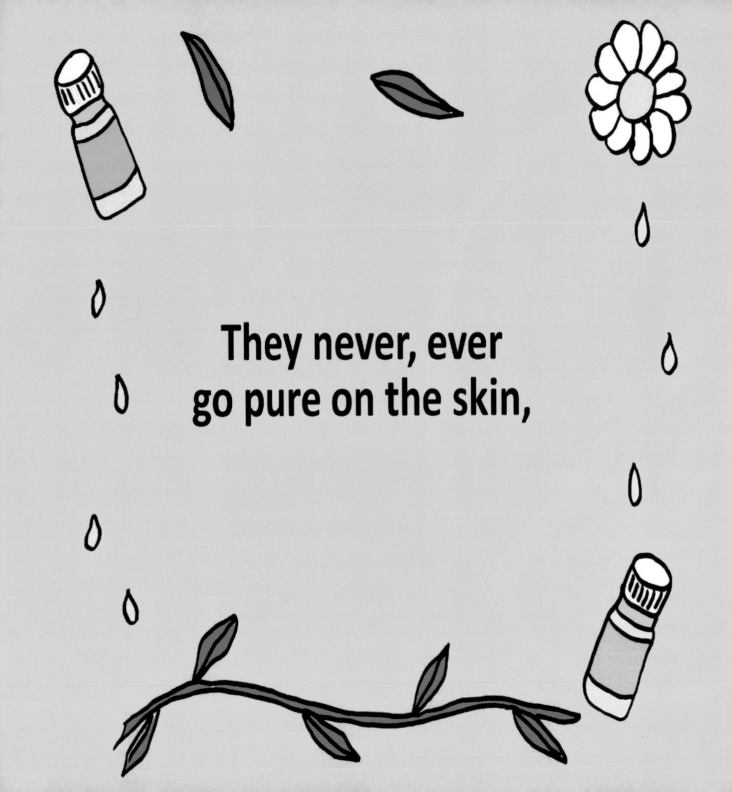

They never, ever
go pure on the skin,

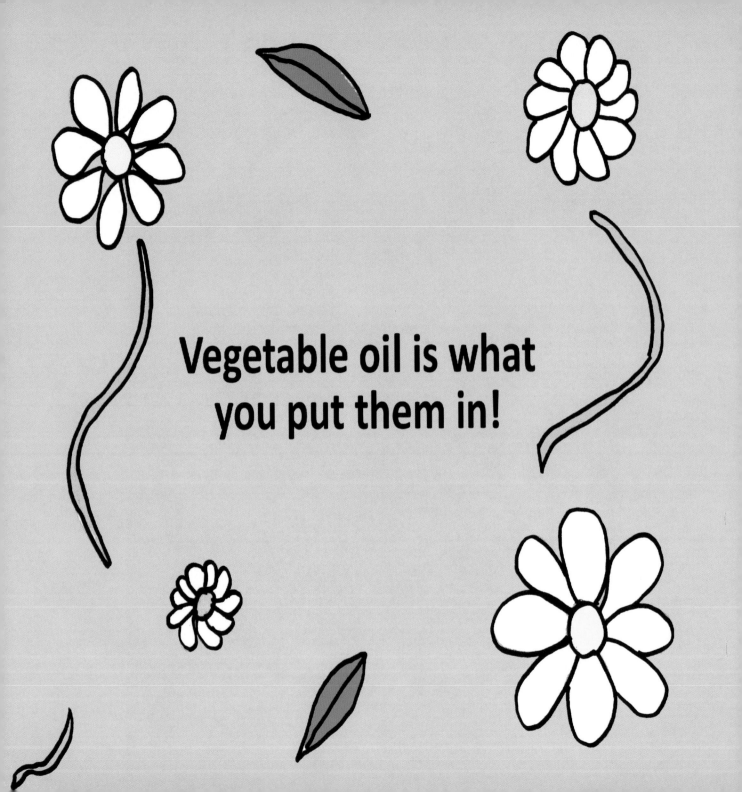

Vegetable oil is what
you put them in!

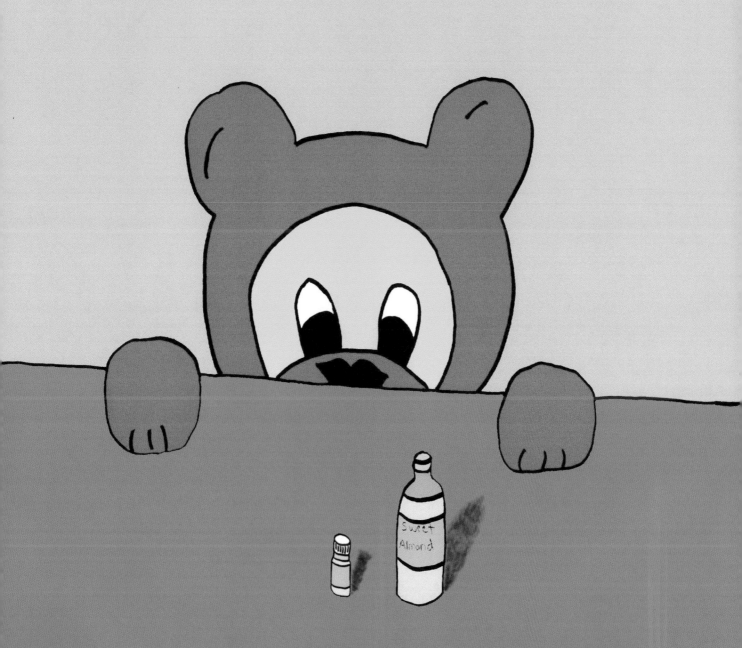

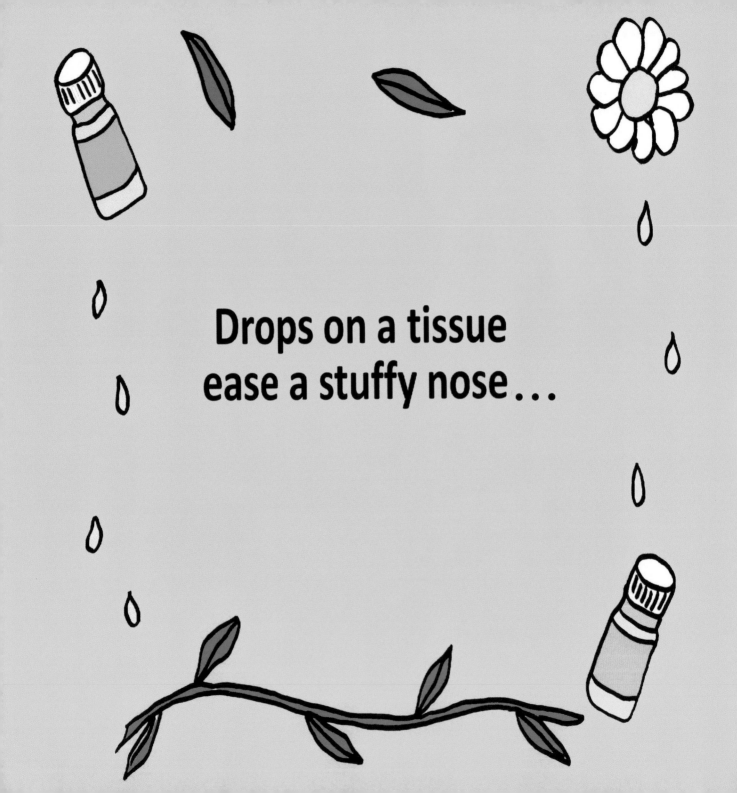

Drops on a tissue
ease a stuffy nose...

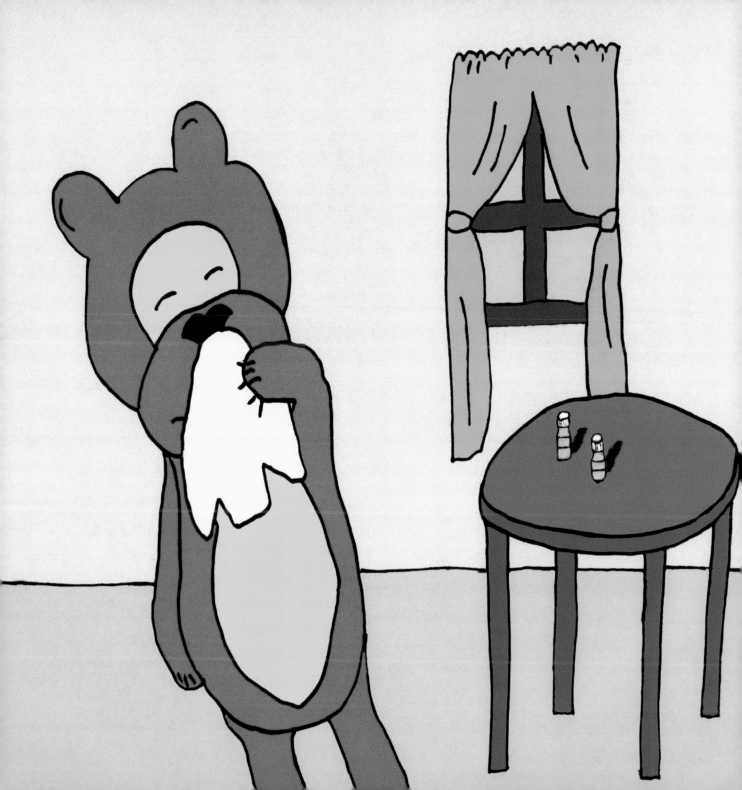

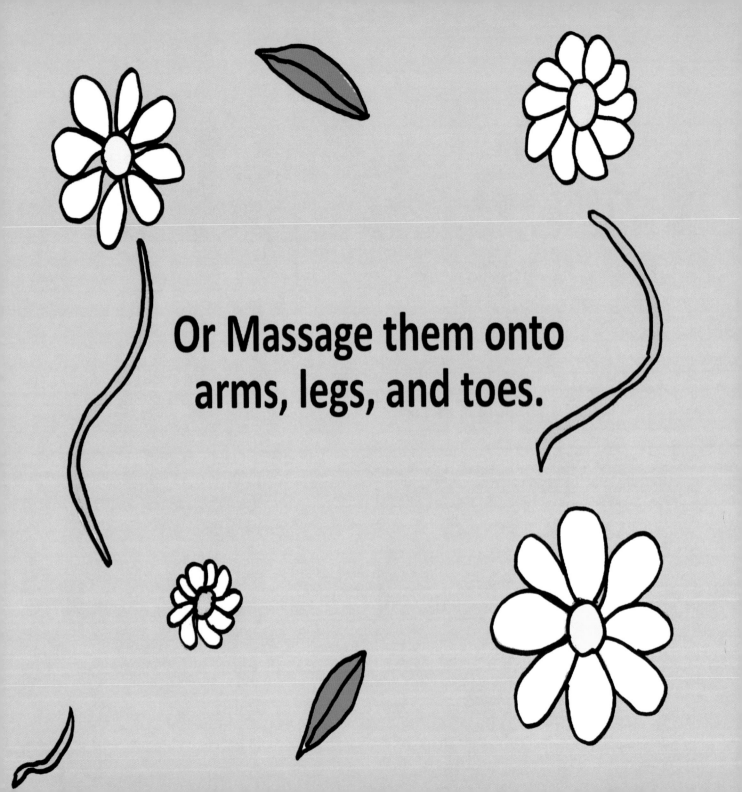

Or Massage them onto
arms, legs, and toes.

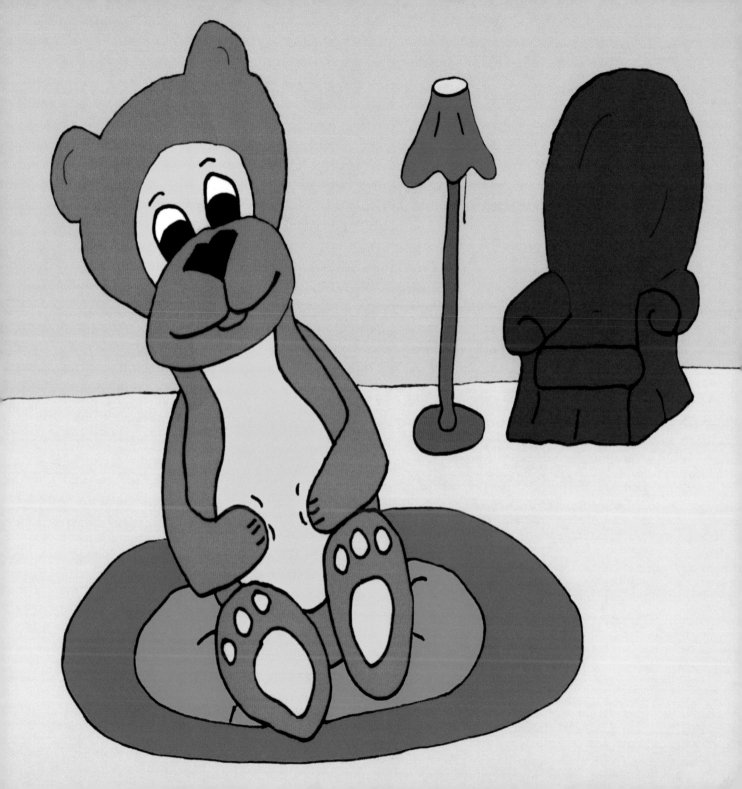

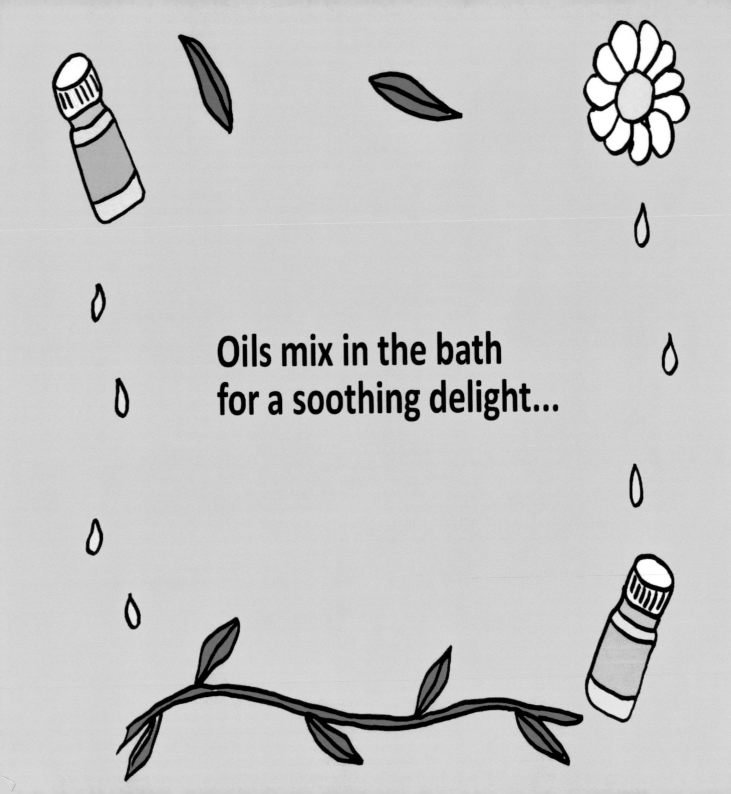

Oils mix in the bath
for a soothing delight...

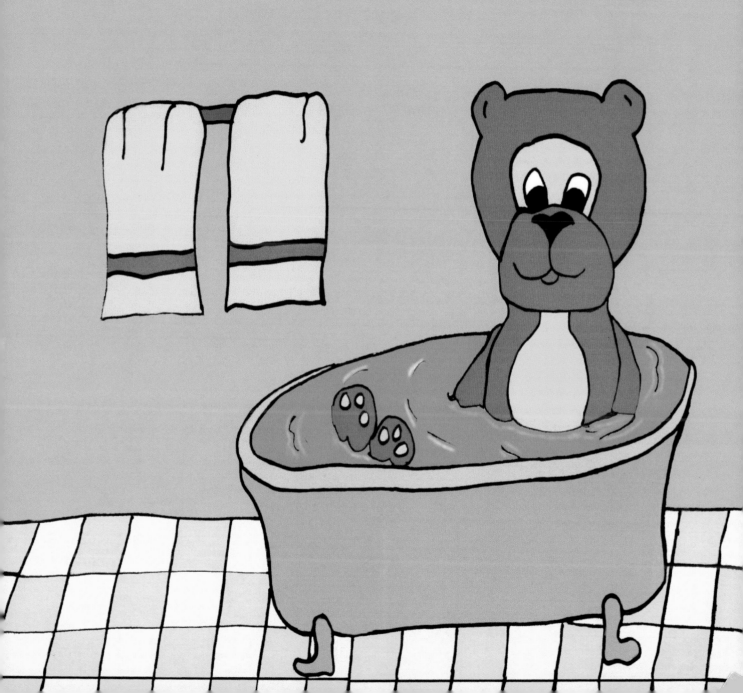

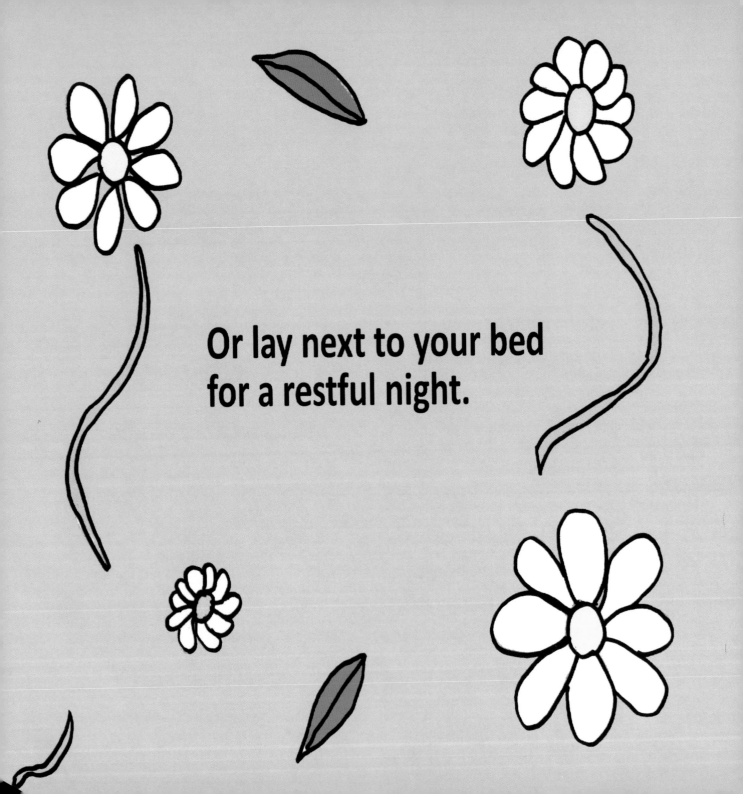

Or lay next to your bed
for a restful night.

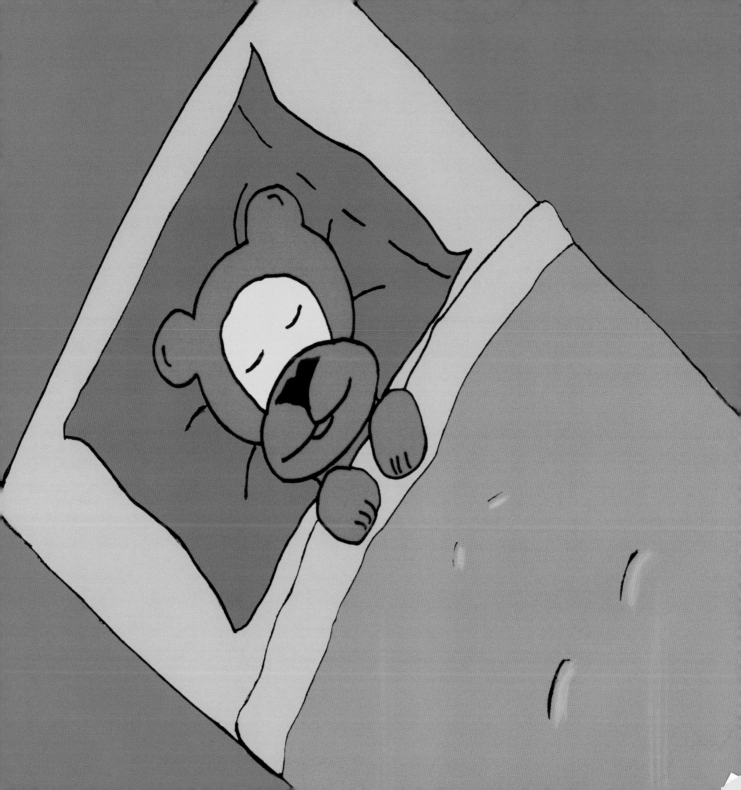